THE DR MOE

RUTH JOCHEMS is
Holland. His interest i
for the disease began
investigations led him to the Dr Moerman Cancer Diet.
He has written several books on the subject of cancer.

DR CORNELIS MOERMAN was a Dutch GP who
began researching 'natural' treatments for cancer in the
1930s. Dr Moerman's diet and therapy have helped to
heal many patients, and modern research is providing
evidence which further backs up his ideas. His therapy is
widely recognised throughout Holland and has recently
received official recognition from the Dutch Ministry of
Health. Dr Moerman died in 1988.

Overcoming Common Problems Series

The ABC of Eating
Coping with anorexia, bulimia and
compulsive eating
JOY MELVILLE

An A–Z of Alternative Medicine
BRENT Q. HAFEN AND KATHRYN J.
FRANDSEN

Arthritis
Is your suffering really necessary?
DR WILLIAM FOX

Being the Boss
STEPHEN FITZSIMON

Birth Over Thirty
SHEILA KITZINGER

Body Language
How to read others' thoughts by their
gestures
ALLAN PEASE

Bodypower
DR VERNON COLEMAN

Calm Down
How to cope with frustration and anger
DR PAUL HAUCK

Comfort for Depression
JANET HORWOOD

Common Childhood Illnesses
DR PATRICIA GILBERT

Complete Public Speaker
GYLES BRANDRETH

Coping with Anxiety and Depression
SHIRLEY TRICKETT

Coping with Depression and Elation
DR PATRICK McKEON

Coping with Stress
DR GEORGIA WITKIN-LANOIL

Coping with Thrush
CAROLINE CLAYTON

**Coping Successfully with Your Child's
Asthma**
DR PAUL CARSON

**Coping Successfully with Your Child's Skin
Problems**
DR PAUL CARSON

**Coping Successfully with Your Hyperactive
Child**
DR PAUL CARSON

**Coping Successfully with Your Irritable
Bowel**
ROSEMARY NICOL

Curing Arthritis Cookbook
MARGARET HILLS

Curing Arthritis – The Drug-free Way
MARGARET HILLS

**Curing Coughs, Colds and Flu – the Drug-
free Way**
MARGARET HILLS

Curing Illness – The Drug-free Way
MARGARET HILLS

Depression
DR PAUL HAUCK

Divorce and Separation
ANGELA WILLANS

The Dr Moerman Cancer Diet
RUTH JOCHEMS

The Epilepsy Handbook
SHELAGH McGOVERN

**Everything You Need to Know about
Adoption**
MAGGIE JONES

**Everything You Need to Know about
Contact Lenses**
DR ROBERT YOUNGSON

**Everything You Need to Know about Your
Eyes**
DR ROBERT YOUNGSON

**Everything You Need to Know about the
Pill**
WENDY COOPER AND TOM SMITH

**Everything You Need to Know about
Shingles**
DR ROBERT YOUNGSON

Overcoming Common Problems Series

Overcoming Common Problems Series

Overcoming Common Problems

THE DR MOERMAN
CANCER DIET

Ruth Jochems

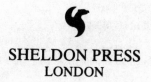

SHELDON PRESS
LONDON

First published in Great Britain 1989
Sheldon Press, SPCK, Marylebone Road, London
NW1 4DU

British Library Cataloguing in Publication Data

Jochems, Ruth
  The Dr Moerman cancer diet
  1. Man. Cancer. Therapy. Diet
  I. Title II. Series
  616.99′40654

  ISBN 0–85969–584–0

Typeset by Deltatype, Ellesmere Port
Printed in Great Britain by Anchor Press Ltd,
Tiptree, Essex

Contents

Publishers' note

This book is published as a contribution to the continuing search for ways in which cancer can be treated. The publishers feel it forms a valuable part of the debate about alternative approaches to cancer, but we do not make any claims about the effectiveness of the Moerman method in curing cancer.

Foreword

About twenty-five years ago my present colleague Dr Ewan Cameron, who was then Chief Surgeon of Vale of Levan Hospital, Loch Lomondside, Scotland, formulated a principle that he thought could be used effectively in the control of cancer. He pointed out that people in good health often recover from cancer, whereas those in poor general health succumb, and suggested that substances that potentiate the body's natural protective mechanisms might well provide some protection against cancer and make a significant contribution to the treatment of cancer. After having tried a number of substances without success, he began in 1971 to give 10 grams of vitamin C per day to patients with advanced cancer, at first by intravenous infusion and then orally. It is now well known that this treatment was beneficial to almost all of the patients and of great value, extending survival time for years, to some of them.

Dr Cornelis Moerman, in The Netherlands, had in fact formulated a similar principle about thirty years earlier. He suggested that persons with good vitality might fight cancer more effectively than those with low vitality, and, in particular, that the vitality of a cancer patient could be greatly increased by adherence to a carefully selected diet. The evidence of his significant success over a fifty-year period is discussed in this book. In the meantime Dr Moerman had trouble with the medical authorities in The Netherlands. I met Dr

Moerman about twenty years ago, and I testified on his behalf when he was under attack. Now, after half a century, he has succeeded in overcoming the opposition. In January 1987 the Ministry of Health in The Netherlands finally granted approval to his treatment.

Dr Moerman's therapy involves eating large amounts of vegetables and fruits, and in particular drinking fruit and vegetable juices in place of water or other beverages. Bakery goods such as white bread, cake, and also foods such as macaroni and spaghetti are forbidden. The intake of sugar is also forbidden, as well as that of meat and animal fat, other than butter. The result is that foods that are poor in vitamins and minerals are not included in the diet, which increases the supply of vitamins and minerals and other important nutrients to the patient. It is my opinion that much of the value of Dr Moerman's therapy results from the high intake of vitamins by the patients.

In the present-day world vitamin supplements are available at a low price, and I believe that Dr Moerman's therapy would be improved by supplementing it with the optimum intake of vitamin C and the other vitamins. In fact, Dr Moerman now recommends a good intake of vitamin C, in addition to the large amount of vitamin C contained in the fruit juices and other foods that he recommends to the patient.

I am glad to recommend this book to cancer patients and their relatives and friends, and to others who want to improve their health by a better selection of foods.

Linus Pauling
22 June 1988

1

Dr Moerman's Great Breakthrough

Saturday 10 January 1987 was a great day in the worldwide fight against cancer. On that day the Dutch Ministry of Health, after thorough research and investigation, gave its official seal of approval to Dr Moerman's breakthrough in the treatment of cancer.

In fact, like most important developments in medicine, the Moerman method hadn't been discovered overnight. It was welcomed in a blaze of publicity, but this sudden fame was really the crowning achievement of more than fifty years work by Dr Moerman, researching, testing and perfecting his great discovery.

All over Holland the media marked the event with interviews with patients who Dr Moerman had successfully cured. There was Mr Kappé, who was told by his doctors that there was nothing they could do for him – he had cancer of the stomach and they couldn't operate. That was eight years ago. Today he's alive and flourishing, thanks to the Moerman method. When they asked the doctor for a comment, all he could say was that perhaps his original diagnosis had been a little cautious.

Then there was the elderly lady who'd had breast cancer. For two years she stuck religiously to Dr Moerman's diet, and now she was completely cured.

Vested interests

A spokesman for the official Dutch cancer research

group wasn't so enthusiastic about these miracles. He argued that these successes didn't prove that the Moerman diet worked, and it was too soon to tell if it really could cure cancer.

This cautious approach is easier to understand when you know a bit of the background. This spokesman was a cancer specialist himself, working on his own idea for a cure, and trying to build his own reputation with it. His approach involved using injections of radio-active iodine, and the money to fund the research was coming from a huge donation of one and a half million dollars, given by the father of an American boy he'd treated. So he had his own reasons for giving Dr Moerman's successes rather a cool reception.

Rivalries between different specialists all competing for money for research cause one set of problems. Huge business interests are also at stake in the search for a cure. Drug companies and manufacturers of surgical instruments all have a vested interest in going through the motions of searching for a cure, pouring money into different 'high-tech' research projects which use their products. A simple self-help therapy like Dr Moerman's, which works through diet, without expensive drugs and treatments, threatens their turnover and their profits.

The scale of the 'cancer industry' was clearly demonstrated recently, when the Managing Director of a major North American drug company revealed that in Europe alone 450 million dollars are spent each year on medicines for cancer and they expect an increase to two billion dollars by 1995.

The largest multi-national drug companies have

cornered the market, and a few giants now control between them 80 per cent of the turnover, while the remaining 20 per cent market share is divided between 95 smaller companies.

New developments

Until recently there were only two major treatments for cancer. Either the patient would be given drugs to try and kill off the tumour (this treatment is called chemo-therapy), or it would be treated with radiation. Both these methods achieved some success in destroying tumours, but the cost to the patient in pain and suffering is enormous. They both have serious side-effects and they wear the patient down both physically and emotionally. Many people find it difficult to go through with a complete course of treatment, and even if they do there is no guarantee that it will be successful.

Recently there have been new developments in research. Nowadays the larger drug companies are researching new drugs using the latest techniques of bio-technology – experimenting with genes and genetic engineering. These new drugs work by reinforcing the body's own defence systems, and scientists now agree that this is their best hope of finding a reliable cure.

The thinking behind these high-tech developments has a lot in common with Dr Moerman's approach. As long ago as the 1930s he had the idea that the natural defence systems and vitality of the human body should be the first focus of attention in the search for a cure for cancer, and that concentrating treatment on the tumour alone could not succeed.

He was years ahead of his time, but now the scientists have begun to catch up. Some doctors have mistrusted his methods because they're so simple, and anyone can use them, but the patients he's cured know that it works.

2
What is Cancer?

The subject of cancer is a daunting one. To begin with, there's such a variety of types of cancer – over 100 different ones – and every case is different. Suppose you've just been told by your doctor that you have a tumour, or you've found a suspicious lump, and you're running through all the worrying possibilities in your mind. The first question is always the same – is the tumour malignant? Tumours can have various causes, but if the doctor says it's malignant, then it's a cancer.

What causes a malignant tumour?

To understand this, you first need to know a bit of background. To begin with – what is a living thing? The simplest kind of living thing can consist of just one cell, and every human being and animal starts out as a single fertilized egg cell. This one cell grows and develops, and the different organs and parts of the body gradually appear.

Every cell in the body forms part of a pattern, and each plays a part which fits smoothly into the running of the whole. A tumour is a group of cells which doesn't fit into this pattern, but sets up an independent system of its own. It's fed by the body, but it doesn't work as part of it.

If a tumour takes over a small quantity of tissue and grows only slowly, it won't have much effect on the rest of the body. This is called a non-malignant tumour. If it grows fast, and bits split off to form other tumours, known as metastases, elsewhere in the body, then it's cancer.

5

Healthy cells get their energy from oxygen, which they produce by a process called oxydation. Cancerous cells get their energy to grow and spread from fermentation. Because of the chemical differences between fermentation and oxydation, healthy cells are much more acid than cancerous ones. So it makes sense to assume that if you can make the cancer cells more acid, more like healthy cells, you'll be able to slow down the growth of the tumour and stop the cancer cells from growing.

Changing the acid balance is the main idea of Dr Moerman's treatment. Then the healing process is continued by strengthening the body's own defence system. Dr Moerman discovered that the body needs eight different substances, the vitamins and minerals found in ordinary food, to do this. If you take them in the right balance they will isolate, break down and eventually destroy the tumour using the defence system. After that, normal tissue can grow back, and the body will heal.

So Dr Moerman's therapy doesn't just focus on the tumour, but it treats it as a symptom of a problem in the whole body, caused by eating the wrong balance of foods. The treatment he prescribes destroys the tumour by treating the whole body. An added benefit of the Moerman method is that the diet which cures cancer will also reinforce your immune system to give you lasting good health. You don't have to be ill to use it – anyone can follow the diet to build up the body's natural defences against disease. It doesn't guarantee eternal life, of course, but it will slow down the ageing process, and protect you against the creeping frailties of old age.

How to help yourseif

When a malignant tumour is diagnosed, you're faced with the daunting task of rebuilding your defences, mental and physical, in order to fight it off. The best boost you can give your body is to talk about the problems, and discuss your fears and feelings with others who've been through it themselves. No-one should have to face questions like 'Will I make it?' on their own. There's now a whole network of support groups, which are usually made up of patients and ex-patients, counsellors and other helpers. Your GP or hospital will be able to put you in touch with a group in your area.

In fact, moral support is the one really crucial element in the healing process. It's especially important during the first few months, when the patient is torn between hope and despair, wondering whether the Moerman method will really work for him or her. But again and again it proves its worth, even with the so-called terminal cases, the ones the doctors have given up hope for.

There are two other questions that often come up when people talk about their worries. The first is the value of early detection. This is certainly very important. The earlier you notice a tumour and start treating it, the quicker the cure. In the early stages secondary tumours have not yet formed, so the body has more strength to fight the tumour.

As far as heredity is concerned, the answer is a definite no. As Dr Moerman shows, cancer is caused by shortages in the diet, so it can't be passed from parent to child.

Hearing the news

Cancer is one of those things that we all want to wish away, and we don't like to think about. If you're confronted by the news that you, or someone close to you, has cancer, it's bound to be a terrible shock. Sometimes it takes weeks, even months, before you recover from the news. Many people find themselves pretending it isn't true – they can't accept the diagnosis. With the exception of Aids, perhaps, no other disease can make you see so clearly the fragility of life.

This phase of shock and denial is followed by a sense of powerlessness and protest – 'Why me?' Then comes depression, and finally you move towards feelings of acceptance.

Cancer patients usually go through a whole range of emotions. Dr Moerman's patients have usually been through chemotherapy and X-ray treatment before they finally come to him, so they've been through a series of different, conflicting feelings – despair, followed by hope of a cure, and then disappointment.

The Moerman regime is by no means a soft option. It *is* strict, but it works, and most people get used to it. Wholewheat bread is nicer than white bread, and brown rice with vegetables and a bit of butter turns out to be very appetizing. Fruit juice instead of coffee and tea can grow on you, and you learn to prefer your food without sugar and salt. At the end of the book you'll find some recipes, to show you what you can do with a little imagination within the restrictions of the diet, and they should inspire you to produce some ideas of your own.

Eating the right food and taking vitamin supplements can never be the whole answer, of course. Your surroundings, and the people around you, are the key to a positive attitude towards yourself and your health, which is the secret weapon for beating cancer. Hope and faith are vital ingredients, and the successes of the Moerman method show that they're always justified.

The chance is there for the taking, and family and friends must support the patient's decision. Relationships with other people are a powerful force, and their help and support will help you win through.

3

First Steps towards
a Cure

In Europe alone a million people die of cancer each year, and some four and a half million undergo some form of treatment for the disease. Of course, no cure is infallible, and the Moerman method doesn't claim to be able to cure every case of cancer. However, a recent survey carried out by a leading cancer research foundation in Holland produced some very encouraging statistics. Of a sample of 150 patients with cancer 60 were cured by using only the Moerman method and a further 55 were cured using the Moerman method when the patients had already received one of the orthodox forms of treatment. This means that more than three-quarters of the patients were cured.

Results like these make you wonder why it took almost 50 years for the therapy to be recognized. To find the answer we must go back to the 1930s, when Dr Moerman began his research.

In the 1930s Dr Moerman was a young, newly qualified doctor, working in a small town in Holland called Vlaardingen. As he worked he became more and more interested not just in diseases and how to cure them, but in good health and how to keep people well. When he examined the patients who came to his surgery, particularly those suffering from cancer, he would look at the whole person, not just the headache or the tumour which had made them come and see him.

Over the years he developed his own ideas about health and disease. His theory was that health is on a spectrum, moving between two poles, like two strong magnets, at either end. Each magnet exerts a pull over your health. He called the two poles vitality and mortality, and as long as vitality, the 'life-force', is stronger than mortality good health is dominant and disease cannot take a hold.

Illness doesn't just strike a healthy person out of the blue. When the body is healthy and strong it can fight off disease. But as soon as its defences are weakened it can't fight back, so viruses and bacteria can invade the body, and in the end it will die.

A sick pigeon

By chance he soon had an opportunity to prove his theory. One day a small boy came to the surgery, and brought his pet pigeon. The bird was ill, and the boy knew that Dr Moerman kept pigeons himself, so he hoped he could save its life.

The pigeon turned out to have a cancerous tumour, and there was nothing he could do for it. After a few weeks' careful nursing it died. As an experiment, though, Dr Moerman took some of the cancer cells from the sick bird, and injected them into a healthy pigeon of his own. This bird showed no ill-effects at all, and this convinced him that cancer cannot be produced in a healthy body.

The body's main defence, which protects it against disease and helps it fight off infection, is the food we eat. If you eat the right food your body will stay healthy, so you can fight off any disease, including cancer cells. If

11

your diet lacks any of the vital elements over a long period, however, you won't be able to fight disease.

This idea was completely new, and it was treated with some suspicion by other cancer experts. The accepted view at that time, which all doctors were taught at medical school, was that tumours are made up of abnormal cells which somehow invade the body. These cells then multiply, and the tumour grows unstopably until it eventually kills the patient. All the research into treatments and cures was focused on the tumour, without taking account of the body's sophisticated defence system and its natural ability to heal itself.

As a result of his own researches, and by observing his patients, Dr Moerman came to the conclusion that this whole approach was wrong, because it was trying to tackle the problem from the wrong end. Treating the tumour on its own might cure some individual patients, but it would never give doctors the key which would solve the whole problem of cancer.

So he changed the starting point, and looked at cancer in a new way. He saw that the vital clue lay in the body's metabolism. This is the name for the chemical changes in the body which maintain life. It not only provides energy for activity, it also keeps the body in good repair – breaking down and carrying away cells which are damaged and useless, and replacing them with new, healthy cells.

The importance of diet

Food is a fuel, and the body runs on food like a car runs on petrol. In order for all these chemical changes to take place as they should the body has to have the right fuel. So metabolism and diet are closely linked to one another.

Dr Moerman found that before cancerous tissue ever appears the metabolism has already become damaged by a diet which, over the years, has not provided all that the body needs. In order to cure cancer, he worked out, you have to start by correcting the metabolism. If the diet and the metabolism are right, the body will be in a state of perfect health.

Some healthy pigeons

By now he had satisfied himself that perfect health is the only defence against cancer, and that the secret of perfect health lies in the diet. In order to discover which elements were necessary in the diet to produce perfect health, once again he turned to his pigeons.

His plan was that what worked for the pigeons might very well work for human beings. Pigeons and people need much the same kind of nutrition, and 24 pigeons eat about as much in a day as one person, which made it possible to calculate the quantities of each substance easily.

Dr Moerman also knew that pigeons burn a huge amount of energy every day flying and keeping their bodies warm. To give you an idea of how much energy they use, a racing pigeon flying in a race may fly as far as 450 miles at a speed of 45 miles an hour. It flaps its wings five times a second, which makes 180,000 wing-beats in one race! To produce all this activity pigeons need to eat a lot of carbohydrates, such as cereals, wheat and rice. These are broken down in the body and stored in the cells. When the body needs to use the stored energy it burns up the carbohydrates. This process is called oxydation. If the diet doesn't contain all the right ingredients oxydation can't take place properly, and instead of burning up carbohydrates to produce energy the body cells begin to ferment. This produces ideal conditions for a cancer to grow. But when you eat the right kind of diet these conditions soon disappear, and the cancer can't survive.

In order to find out what the best diet was he kept his pigeons in separate compartments for a while. He varied their diet by adding or leaving out particular foods, and noted the results.

To begin with he gave all his pigeons the same food for a while, so that their basic state of health would be the same when the experiment began. Then he divided them into two groups, and gave them different food. First he gave one group yeast, which contains lots of vitamin B, in their drinking water, while the other group got ordinary water. Then he gave the first group wheat as well as yeast, and fed the second group on breadcrumbs.

After a few weeks the first group were perfectly healthy, but the second group had become weak, and got tired very easily. Dr Moerman worked out that the lack of proper nutrition in the breadcrumbs meant these pigeons couldn't burn energy properly, and that was why they got so tired.

Over the years he tested lots of different foods, containing different vitamins and minerals. He discovered that there are eight elements which are essential for good heath. These are:

Vitamin A	Citric Acid
Vitamin B	Iodine
Vitamin C	Sulphur
Vitamin E	Iron

If the pigeons didn't get all these eight elements in their diet they developed serious health problems. They began to look scruffy and listless, they couldn't fly so far or for so long, and some of them began to show obvious signs of illness within a very short time.

So he researched and observed the pigeons, and took notes about their health, fitness and stamina, until he had enough evidence to prove that these eight elements were vital for healthy cells, and a lack of them was directly responsible for the birds' ill health.

4

The Vital Ingredients of Good Health

The Eight Substances

Each of these vitamins and minerals plays an important part in keeping the body healthy. They have their own functions, and they interact in the body, working together in the right balance to produce perfect health. In order to understand Dr Moerman's diet it's vital to know what they do and what foods they're found in.

Vitamin A

Vitamin A protects the skin, and the mucus tissues such as the gums. It's also important for the eyes – it prevents night-blindness and helps weak eyesight. In pregnant women it's vital for the growth of the foetus, and it helps prevent acne in teenagers.

It's found in milk, eggs, cod-liver oil, butter, and in many vegetables, for example, carrots, tomatoes and spinach.

Vitamin B

Vitamin B is in fact a whole group of vitamins, known as the B complex. The different vitamins in it are known by different names or numbers. It includes *thiamin* (B1), *riboflavin* (B2), *nicotinamide*, *folic acid*, *pantothenic acid*, *pyridoxin* (B6), *biotin* and the *cobalamins* (B12).

Thiamin (B1) is necessary for the metabolism of carbohydrates, especially in the nervous system. A shortage of thiamin leads to beriberi – inflammation of the nerves, with muscle weakness and heart fatigue.

The best sources are seeds, such as natural rice and wheat germ, but it's also found in milk, fruit and yeast.

Riboflavin (B2) is essential to help the cells breathe properly. Brittle nails and chapped hands and lips are all signs of a deficiency.

It is found in milk, eggs, fresh vegetables and yeast.

Pyridoxin (B6) is an important member of the B group. It plays a part in the metabolism of the protein in the diet, and it produces a substance called properdin, part of the body's natural immune system, which destroys bacteria and viruses in the blood. A shortage of pyridoxin affects the central nervous system, and causes sleeplessness, irritability and mood changes.

It's found in yeast, green vegetables and cereals.

Biotin is essential for growth, for producing enzymes, which are necessary for digesting food, and for maintaining the body's acid balance. Skin problems, including greasy skin and hair, are caused by a lack of biotin in the diet.

Yeast and egg yolk are good sources of biotin.

Vitamin B12 is in fact a range of substances which are vital for healthy blood. If you don't have enough, it causes anaemia and tiredness.

17

Egg yolk is particularly rich in B12.

Vitamin C

Vitamin C is the best-known of all the vitamins. It's a 'multi-purpose' vitamin – it's vital for cell metabolism, it helps the body get rid of poisons, it protects it against the harmful nitrates in cheese and meat, it helps it absorb iron, it dissolves cholesterol, it stimulates the cells which produce interferon, which fights off virus infections, and it protects the body against cancer. Taken daily it strengthens the immune system and reinforces the body's natural ability to heal itself.

Dr Moerman isn't the only cancer specialist to prescribe vitamin C for his patients. A doctor working in Scotland, Dr Cameron, was the first to experiment with it. His patients took 10 grams a day for a long time, and he achieved some good results. And of course Dr Linus Pauling, who has won two Nobel Prizes, is famous for his work in the fight against cancer, and who has written the foreword for this book, has always been a firm advocate of vitamin C.

Dr Moerman met Professor Pauling when he was giving a lecture in the United States, and Professor Pauling invited him to come to San Francisco to see his work, as a token of 'his sincere appreciation of Moerman's great contribution to the solution of the cancer problem'.

A lack of vitamin C causes scurvy – weak bones and muscles, bleeding gums and increased risk of infection.

Vitamin E

Vitamin E is important for fertility and for slowing down

18

the effect of ageing all over the body. It's vital during pregnancy, it helps produce sex hormones in both men and women and the nervous system can't work without it. It helps build body tissue, muscle fibre and blood vessels.

Vitamin E is also essential for metabolism and 'breathing' in the cells. It's an anti-oxidant, which means it prevents fats from being destroyed in the body by oxygen, and it protects the body against cancer.

If you don't get enough vitamin E it can cause brown 'liver spots' on your skin as you get older. It can also lead to infertility and miscarriages.

Vitamin E is found in wheatgerm, whole grain cereals and vegetable oils.

Citric acid

The lemon is a very important fruit in the Moerman diet. As well as being a rich source of vitamin C it also contains citric acid and a vitamin called citrin, also known as vitamin P. Citrin helps the blood flow freely through even the tiniest blood vessels, the capillaries, which deliver blood to the skin. A shortage of citrin clogs up the capillaries, and causes swollen legs, ankles and feet.

Citric acid also helps the blood flow, as it takes water from the body tissues to thin the blood. By doing this it prevents fermentation in the cells, it protects the body from blood clots, and it regulates the acid balance.

Iodine

Iodine is a mineral, one of the substances which the body needs in small quantities, but which are vital for good health.

It regulates the thyroid, which produces growth hormones. The most important of these hormones is called thyroxine, and it controls the basic rate of metabolism in the body, by making the cells absorb oxygen. If you don't get enough iodine the cells can't get enough oxygen to breathe, so they begin to ferment.

Most people get all the iodine they need from drinking water, but in some places, such as Derbyshire and parts of Switzerland, the water doesn't contain enough. Until the value of iodine was discovered doctors were baffled by the number of cases of goitre and stunted growth, two of the problems caused by iodine deficiency, they diagnosed. Nowadays iodine is added to table salt, so everyone gets enough in their diet.

Sulphur

The importance of sulphur can be summed up by saying that it helps the body get rid of any poisonous materials. It's also necessary for the mitochodrics, which are microscopic organisms in the cells, which produce energy. Sulphur and iodine work together to ensure that the cells breathe properly.

Iron

The human body needs iron to produce red blood cells. Lack of iron causes anaemia, which makes you lose your appetite and feel constantly tired, and you fall victim to one infection after another.

Vitamin D

As well as these eight substances, the human body also needs vitamin D for good health. Vitamin D is necessary for the body to absorb the calcium and phosphorus in the food we eat. It builds bones, especially in young children, and protects the bones against weakening diseases, such as rickets and osteoporosis. Cancer patients with a tumour on or near their bones need a good supply of vitamin D.

The best source is fish oil, particularly cod-liver oil.

The Moerman Theory

Each of the eight substances plays a part in keeping the body in a state of perfect health, and you can't be healthy unless you have enough of each one. If one is in short supply the body can't compensate for it by using something else, but instead it will begin to lose all the other substances. Their combined action has three main effects on the human body:

- The acid balance remains normal
- The trigger for disease, which is present as a virus in cancer patients, cannot penetrate into the bloodstream
- Body tissue is renewed and replaced properly

When the body doesn't contain enough of these eight substances, the following problems appear:

- The acid level shifts away from acidity towards an alkaline state, and this results in more fermentation and less oxydation – in other words the cells can't absorb enough oxygen
- The harmful virus penetrates the bloodstream and begins to spread

- The new tissue which the body produces is abnormal – if it's examined under a microscope it clearly doesn't have the same structure and characteristics as other tissue.

When you follow the Moerman diet and the eight substances become active:

- The acid level returns towards acid
- The virus diminishes and in the end is totally destroyed
- Normal tissue grows again

This is the basis of the Moerman therapy.

5

Symptoms and Successes

Once he had come to this conclusion, and backed it up with thorough scientific evidence, Dr Moerman began to examine patients who came to see him with cancer with special care. He observed that they often seemed to have certain other symptoms, which were definitely caused by a lack of one or more of these eight elements in their diet.

Some Symptoms of Vitamin Shortage

1. *Dry skin*, which has lost its elasticity and tends to wrinkle easily, suggests a long-term shortage of vitamn A. Dr Moerman also noticed that the soles of the feet tend to build up hard skin and become very calloused, and the skin becomes 'scaly', and makes the patient look grey and ill.

2. *The mucus tissue* – the parts of the body which are usually moist – often show symptoms which show a lack of riboflavin (vitamin B2). For example, the tongue may be unusually bright red.

3. *The corners of the mouth may become chapped*, and this too is caused by a shortage of riboflavin. It's often a problem for elderly people.

4. *Red spots and scaly skin around the nostrils* are also

23

caused by a shortage of riboflavin. Riboflavin is vital for healthy cell respiration and growth, so a lack of it in the diet shows up all over the body in many different ways.

5. *Dull nails and rough, chapped hands* are also caused by insufficient riboflavin.

6. *A brown, furry coating on the tongue* is an indication of a lack of nicotinamide, one of the B complex vitamins.

7. *Lifeless hair.* If your hair is dull and dry, or if it starts to fall out more than usual, it probably means there's a shortage of pantothenic acid, another of the B complex, in your diet.

8. *Gums which bleed* when you brush your teeth are a sign of lack of vitamin C.

9. *Bruising easily.* If a slight knock gives you a black bruise, it suggests a shortage of vitamin C.

10. *Slow healing of wounds* and

11. *'Jelly-like' tissue* forming in a wound after an operation or a deep cut are signs of lack of vitamin C.

12. *Feeling exhausted for no reason* are all signs of a lack of vitamin E. This vitamin is essential to let the cells digest and breathe properly. It's sometimes called the 'old age vitamin', because older people often don't have enough of it in their diet.

13. *A pale complexion* indicates that you're short of iron and cobalt.

14. *A craving for sour foods*, such as lemons and pickles, suggests that there's not enough acid in the body, so its acid balance is wrong.

15. *Feeling apathetic and listless* suggests a lack of all the eight vital elements, and shows that your body's defence system is weakened.

16. *Tiredness* is also caused by a shortage of iodine and sulphur in the diet. These two elements play an important part in helping the cells absorb oxygen. Without them oxydation can't take place properly, and this has two harmful results. The body can't produce enough energy, so you feel tired all the time, and the cells begin to ferment, and as we've seen, that can be the first step towards cancer.

17. *Sudden weight loss* is caused by a lack of sulphur in the diet. Sulphur is also necessary to convert food into substances which the body can use.

All these symptoms are warning signs that something is wrong with the metabolism, and it isn't getting the eight substances it needs. Because the eight substances are all necessary for the cells to breathe properly, each one of these symptoms shows that the body isn't able to absorb the oxygen it needs. Everyone needs oxygen to live – if you stopped breathing and held your breath you'd be dead within a matter of minutes – and every cell in your body needs oxygen to live and breathe.

So these symptoms aren't just signs that you're under the weather. To fight off diseases, including cancer, you have to be in perfect health. Anything less means your body could be heading for danger.

The seventeen symptoms are all caused by faulty nutrition, and that doesn't happen overnight. It's the result of eating the wrong food over a long period – perhaps many years. But once your body has sent the danger signals you can put the damage right with the Moerman diet.

Dr Moerman's First Success

His careful observation of his pigeons and his patients, and his painstaking identification of the eight substances and seventeen symptoms, laid the foundation of Dr Moerman's therapy. His next step was to make a brave leap from theory to practice. He needed to find a patient who would agree to be a 'human guinea-pig', who he could treat according to his new ideas and see if they would work on humans.

In December 1939 a man called Mr Brinkman came to see him. The doctor had diagnosed a tumour in his stomach. He had been all set to have an operation to remove it, but when the surgeon began to operate he discovered that the tumour had spread to his groin and legs, so it was too late for surgery to help him. Mr Brinkman had nothing to lose, so he put his life in Dr Moerman's hands.

Over the next year he ate oranges and lemons 'by the truckload', he said later, until he was up to his eyes in vitamin C. But it worked! When the year was up he was cured, and the first patient to be healed by the Moerman method lived to be 90 years old.

6

The Immune System

Spurred on by his success with Mr Brinkman, Dr Moerman went on to develop his ideas in more detail. He already knew that the body has to be perfectly healthy to fight off invading bacteria and viruses which cause disease. Next, he turned his attention to the immune system, the natural defence mechanism which protects the body.

Many doctors now recognize that the immune system is the key to good health. After all, it makes sense to do all you can to strengthen this natural process and help the body help itself, rather than inventing new drugs to kill each individual germ. The importance of the immune system has been brought into tragic focus by the arrival of Aids, which shows all too clearly what happens when the immune system is destroyed. The newest research shows that the way forward with many diseases, including Aids and cancer, may well lie in encouraging the natural healing of the immune system.

The Immune System

The immune system is the name given to the way the human body protects itself against illness. You can picture it as being like an army fighting off invaders, and it uses two different kinds of weapons.

The white corpuscles, which are found in the blood-stream, are the first weapon. When they find harmful bacteria or viruses, which cause disease, in the body they absorb and 'digest' them. The second weapon is provided by substances in the body which protect it against the effects of these harmful bacteria, so they can't get a foothold and multiply in the body.

The body is producing these weapons all the time. When the temperature in the body rises, white blood cells and immune substances can be produced more quickly. This is what produces the high temperature when you have a fever – caused by your body fighting back against disease.

As well as 'digesting' harmful bacteria, the white blood cells have another important function. Every day, in the natural course of events, lots of cells and tissue die, and are no longer needed. If they stayed in the body they would build up and rot, and eventually poison it. The white cells break down this dead matter, and help the body get rid of it.

To do this, the body needs to produce one and a half million white blood cells every second. The bone marrow, the spleen and the glands are all involved in this enormous production process, so they need a constant supply of the right vitamins and minerals to nourish them. If they don't get enough, the body can't produce enough white blood cells and the immune system is weakened.

The Nervous System

The nervous system controls all the functions of the body. It includes the brain, the spine, and all the other processes that keep us alive. Some of its functions are under our conscious control. For example, when you decide to stretch out your hand and pick up a pencil, the stages of the process – all the muscle movements and the decision – are consciously controlled. All the other functions are the job of the *autonomic* nervous system, which controls all the activities we don't need to think about. It regulates the heart, the circulation of the blood, the water levels in the body, the workings of the hormones, all the body secretions, breathing, digestion, and metabolism. The autonomic nervous system is itself divided into two parts, the *sympathetic* and the *parasympathetic*, which balance each other out.

In looking at the metabolism it's the sympathetic system we're interested in, because it controls the breakdown of foods, and the increase in cells by division. And the sympathetic system doesn't only play a role in controlling healthy cells, which get their energy from oxygen. When a cell has lost its ability to use oxygen, and starts to get its energy from fermentation it is the sympathetic nervous system which should activate the body's rejection system, to make it dispose of the damaged cell. If the metabolism is healthy this can be done easily, but if the immune system has been weakened the fermenting cells will be able to increase unhindered, and the sympathetic nervous system won't work properly.

To restore the nervous system the first priority is to restore the correct acid balance in the body. As the body moves toward a more acid state the cells can begin to take in oxygen again, and the sympathetic nervous system can take control over the cells again, and regulate cell division properly.

The Moerman diet is designed to provide all the ingredients the immune system needs to work properly. This is vital to prevent cancer. If your body isn't cleaned out by white blood cells damaged cells and tissue will be left, which don't absorb their full amount of oxygen. This is very dangerous, because it can herald the growth of a cancer.

Although Dr Moerman's ideas seem now to be sensible and logical, based on respect for the body's own sophisticated methods for healing itself, he came up against a lot of resistance from other doctors.

In the 1930s the accepted view was that cancer was a disease that affected particular parts of the body, producing a tumour, and the tumour was the problem. So when doctors looked for a cure they concentrated on the tumour, because this was where all their training had taught them to look. Chemotherapy and X-ray treatment were developed, and they had some success, but they produced terrible side-effects on the patients – their hair fell out, and they felt constantly depressed, sick and exhausted. Both treatments involve bombarding the tumour with very powerful weapons, so it's hardly surprising that they have devastating effects on healthy tissue too.

Perhaps one of the reasons why other doctors were so suspicious of Dr Moerman's ideas might be that his cure was so simple. It had no side-effects, anyone could use it and it worked. His cure also showed that the other doctors had been working on the problem from the wrong end, and that can't have made him popular in medical circles either.

Lately, however, after so many years of isolation, Dr

Moerman's ideas have begun to be echoed by the most famous scientists working on a cure for cancer. Many people are now interested in the idea of treating the whole person, rather than concentrating on symptoms. And Dr Moerman can back up his theory with an impressive list of people he's cured.

Dr Linus Pauling, the Nobel prize winner world famous for his work to find a cure for cancer, called one of Dr Moerman's books 'a great contribution to the solution of the cancer problem'. Dr Pauling is also convinced that vitamin C provides a vital clue to the cure.

Other prominent scientists working on a cure have begun to agree with Dr Moerman's argument that the old view is wrong, and they have carried out experiments to show that cancer develops when the body's physical defences are weakened.

Recently a lot of research has been carried out into how the immune system works, as part of the search for a cure for Aids. The latest findings support Dr Moerman's theory that a healthy immune system can fight off cancer. Doctors also agree that fermentation in the cells is a vital factor in the development of cancer. Time and again the most modern research backs up Dr Moerman's theories, even though they were dismissed as nonsense all those years ago.

A few years later, evidence to back up Dr Moerman's ideas appeared from an unexpected source. When statistics were published for the number of cases of cancer in Holland between 1940 and 1950, they told an interesting story.

The figures were collected by another doctor, who was

31

writing an article about the connection between health and prosperity, to see if the amount of money people had to spend on food made them more or less healthy. The figures showed that between 1942 and 1945 the number of cases of cancer fell dramatically. After the Second World War was over the number began to rise again.

One of the reasons for this was food rationing. Instead of the white bread people had eaten before the war, they could only get wholemeal and rye bread; white sugar, coffee and tea weren't available at all; butter was scarce and margarine production stopped completely; spirits, wine and beer became luxuries and instead people drank fruit juice; and meat was very scarce. So everyone was eating exactly the sort of diet which Dr Moerman advised to prevent and cure cancer – no white bread, fats, meat or alcohol, lots of fruit, vegetables and wholemeal bread. When the war was over and rationing ended, people returned to their old eating habits, and the number of new cancer cases increased again.

Dr Moerman was born in 1893, and in 1985 he celebrated the 55th anniversary of his great work. He died in 1988, in his 96th year – an excellent advertisement for his prescription for healthy living!

7

How the Cure Works

Dr Moerman's natural cure divides the healing process into three stages:

- Stopping the growth of the tumour
- Walling off the tumour by encapsulation
- Breaking the tumour down

To make the method work the patient needs three things:

- The diet

- The vitamin supplements

- A will of iron, to stick to the diet and take the supplements religiously

If you've got all three, you can cure yourself! Here are some case histories, to show how successful it can be.

Mrs Schmidt, from Rotterdam, had breast cancer, with secondary tumours in her lungs. Her doctors thought it was too late to operate, as the tumours were so far advanced. She turned to Dr Moerman, and tried his natural cure as her last hope. After five months of his treatment the tumour in her breast had stopped growing. The tumour had become walled off, which meant it could be removed by surgery. Meanwhile the tumours in her lungs had broken down and disappeared.

Mr Reuben, from The Hague, had a skin cancer under his chin. He had an operation, but the tumour returned, and after a whole series of unsuccessful operations he decided to let Dr Moerman treat him. Eight months later, the cancer had completely disappeared.

Mr Koenig had a dangerous growth in his intestines. He underwent five courses of radium therapy, but to no avail. The tumour grew to the size of a coconut, and he was told he was incurable. He went to Dr Moerman, and put his life in his hands. The treatment worked, and Mr Koenig was cured.

I could go on and on with a list of Dr Moerman's successes. In Holland some 42 doctors won't use any other method to treat people with cancer, and you can get his diet in almost any hospital.

This is an amazing breakthrough, when you consider the resistance of orthodox doctors to Dr Moerman's discoveries, and how reluctant they were to be convinced. Not so the patients, who knew that thanks to Dr Moerman and his simple, natural cure, they now had a new lease of life, after the traditional doctors had given up all hope for them.

The Regime of Supplements

As Dr Moerman worked on his ideas his fame began to spread. Although the doctors and scientists were still concentrating on cures for tumours, more and more people who had cancer themselves heard about his successes, and wanted to see if his therapy would work for them.

So he began to ask himself some more questions about how to break down and destroy cancers:

- What is the best possible balance between the different vitamins and minerals?
- What quantities of each vitamin and mineral do you need to take each day?
- Is there anything else you should take as well?

To help him answer these questions he tried out different amounts of vitamins and minerals on his patients, and he noticed the effects not just on their tumours, but also on the other symptoms listed in Chapter 5, which are signs of a lack of vitamins and minerals.

He noticed that if he gave his patients a small amount of vitamin A, for example, it had practically no effect. However, when he increased the dose little by little the callouses disappeared, the patient's skin got clearer and the tumour stopped growing. He found that the most effective dose was as high as 50,000 International Units a day, rising to 100,000 in some cases. He also saw that tablets which included some vitamin D were especially effective, as it helps the body absorb vitamin A.

Dr Moerman tried out his new cure on patients with varicose ulcers, a painful complication of varicose veins, and one which can be dangerous. They followed the Moerman diet, and ate lots of oranges and lemons, which contain ascorbic acid, citric acid and vitamin C. The patients also took generous doses of vitamins A and E, and iodine, and within six weeks their ulcers were completely healed.

35

Over the years he examined the effects of all the vitamins and minerals he knew were necessary to keep the immune system healthy, and gradually he began to piece together the answers to his questions. Little by little he developed his diet, which provides all the body needs to stay fit and healthy, and just as importantly forbids foods which damage the body and prevent good, nutritious foods from being used properly. This diet can be used by anyone who wants to take responsibility for their own good health and protect themself against cancer.

For his patients who had cancer he also developed a regime of vitamin supplements, because they needed huge doses to destroy their tumours. Often the patients who came to him for help had been written off by their doctors because their tumours were too advanced for surgery, and once the disease had spread this far the body would need a lot of help to fight back.

Vitamin C

As he continued to work with cancer patients he noticed that they were often listless – they had no energy or enthusiasm for life. But as soon as they began to eat oranges and lemons in larger quantities, and take daily supplements of vitamin C, their whole outlook on life changed, and their attitude became much more positive. The ascorbic acid allowed the cells to absorb more oxygen, and this automatically increases the body's vitality.

Even more important, these high doses of vitamin C had a dramatic effect on the tissues around the tumour, which, trapped in almost impenetrably dense scar tissue was isolated, and couldn't grow any further.

The idea of drinking gallons of lemon juice may sound very daunting, but Dr Moerman noticed that all his patients had a craving for sour foods. Even people who had previously loved sweets and chocolate began to demand oranges and lemons, as if their bodies were suddenly telling them what they needed to be healthy again.

The benefits of lots of citrus fruits – oranges and lemons, limes and grapefruit, cannot be stressed too often. Citric acid is important because it thins the blood and helps it flow properly, and it also cuts down the levels of cholesterol in the blood, which can cause heart attacks. It also prevents the dangerous fermentation process, which provides the conditions where a tumour can grow.

Citric acid also prevents the tissues retaining water. This is very important, because cancerous tissue contains a lot of excess water, and this in turn helps more cancerous tissue to grow. For this reason tea and coffee, which encourage the body to retain water, are forbidden on the Moerman diet.

Citric acid also keeps the blood and tissues acid, and prevents the body from becoming too alkaline. If this happens, the cells ferment and cancers can grow. Keeping the body acid is especially important to prevent or cure skin cancer.

Dose

Dr Moerman recommends 1250 mg vitamin C every day, rising to 10 g for serious cases of cancer.

Vitamin E

As well as listlessness, many of Dr Moerman's patients complained that they felt tired all the time. He found that vitamin E was the best cure for this, as it affects the pituitary gland, which regulates energy levels all round the body, and it makes the heart and the blood vessels work more efficiently.

Vitamin E was always thought to increase the sex-drive, but Dr Moerman found this didn't happen. He did notice, however, that a good supply of vitamin E is vital to help the liver do its work properly, removing poisons from the blood-stream.

Dose

Dr Moerman prescribes 50 mg vitamin E daily.

Iron

Another problem for people with cancer is anaemia. The answer is to take an iron supplement. As well as curing the anaemia, and making patients feel more active and energetic, iron helps the oxydation process, which increases the body's vitality.

Dose

One iron tablet every day.

Sulphur

A tumour in the stomach or the intestines slows down the cells' 'breathing', so they can't burn energy properly, and this means the body can't digest food. A healthy digestion is very important, because without it the body can't get the full benefit from the food you eat. So it's vital to help the digestion all you can. Sulphur is very important, as it helps destroy tumours in the stomach.

Dose

Half a gram purified sulphur first thing in the morning and last thing at night.

Iodine

Dr Moerman also prescribes his patients a small amount of iodine. However, iodine should always be used sparingly, as it can weaken the red blood-cells, and it should never be taken by people with anaemia. He only uses it to ensure that his patients' diet doesn't leave them short of it, as it's vital for the thyroid and the growth hormones.

Water-soluble and fat-soluble vitamins

When the doses of the different vitamins for the Dr Moerman diet were worked out one very important factor in deciding the various amounts was how the vitamins are stored in the body. If you take in more vitamin C than your body needs your body can't store the surplus until it needs it, so it's passed out through the kidneys. This means that you have to take some every day to make sure you have enough, but there's no risk of a surplus building up to dangerous levels. On the other hand other vitamins, such as vitamin A, can be stored in the liver. The difference is that some vitamins are fat-soluble, which means they dissolve in fat and *can* be stored, and others are water-soluble, which means they dissolve in water and get passed out in the urine – they *can't* be stored.

The most important fat-soluble vitamins are A, D, E and K, and they can be stored over a long period. To encourage this you should always eat cold-pressed olive oil or sunflower oil on your salads, to help the vitamins dissolve so the body can use them.

The water-soluble vitamins are C, B1 (thiamin), B2 (riboflavin), B6 (pyridoxin), B12, biotin, pantothenic acid, nicotinic acid and folic acid. None of these except B12 can be stored, so a shortage will show up quickly if there isn't enough in your diet.

Sources of Vitamins and Minerals

This is a summary of the best food sources of the vitamins and minerals that keep the immune system healthy. If you're following the Dr Moerman diet, however, you must check that each food is permitted. This is only a general guide.

Vitamin A

Carrots, green-leaf vegetables such as spinach and kale, tomatoes, butter, milk, apricots, rose-hips, peaches, parsley.

Vitamin B Complex

Asparagus, broccoli, nuts, egg-yolk, cereals, brown rice, milk, tomatoes, parsley .

Vitamin C

Fresh fruit, especially oranges, grapefruit, rose-hips, blackcurrants, leaf vegetables, brussels sprouts, green cabbage, cauliflower, parsley, turnips, onions, leeks, french beans, tomatoes, cucumber, celery.

Vitamin E

Wheat germ, green peas, olive oil, wholemeal bread (see p. 51), egg yolk, nuts.

And in smaller quantities in milk, butter, spinach and cereals.

Citric acid

All citrus fruits – oranges, lemons, limes, grapefruit etc.

Iodine

Lemons, cauliflower, turnips, brown rice, rye, wheat germ, wholemeal bread, milk, butter, egg yolk.

Sulphur

Onions, garlic, strawberries, gooseberries, green peas, cheese, rye, barley, oats, brown rice, wheat, walnuts, leeks, sea-salt, celery, melons, olives, egg yolk, hazel-nuts, almonds.

Iron

Rye, wheat germ, egg yolk, brussels sprouts, nuts, barley, oats, peas, berries – bilberries, blackberries, cranberries, strawberries, gooseberries, red and black-currants – leaf vegetables, asparagus, beetroot, parsley, tomatoes, honey, brown rice, radishes, wholemeal bread, buckwheat, yeast.

8

Introduction to the Diet

The Moerman diet isn't just for people with cancer. It's carefully worked out to strengthen the body's immune system and balance the metabolism, so it will keep you healthy as effectively as it cures. And surely it makes sense to prepare your defences rather than waiting until your body's attacked to fight back?

If you feel constantly tired or you're always a bit under the weather, or if you have any of the symptoms listed in Chapter 5, it's a sure sign that your immune system and your metabolism aren't getting the fuel they need for peak performance. When you try the Moerman diet you'll find it involves sacrifices at first, but gradually you'll feel fitter and healthier than you have for years. Many people find that minor health problems they've had for a long time, that they'd always put down to getting older, or they'd just learned to live with, disappear, leaving them feeling younger and more energetic.

As you get older, your body's vitality naturally tends to decline and weaken, so it becomes more and more important with the passing of the years to boost your vitality. Some old people seem to glow with health, and they aren't troubled by the niggling aches and pains that others take for granted. That's what a healthy diet can do.

Another important factor in the fight against cancer is

your attitude of mind, and this is especially true as you get older. If cancer has become established in the body and the patient has a fatalistic attitude, determined that they won't recover, then even with the Moerman method the healing benefits could be cancelled out by the patient's own approach to life.

The body is ruled by the mind, and someone who doesn't have the will to live can never help their body heal itself. Elderly men, for example, often fall victim to cancer of the prostate, and instead of fighting against it they give in to illness, and never recover.

The importance of the right nutrition, especially as you grow older, can't be emphasized too often. Older people tend to eat less than they did when they were younger, and that should be reason enough to make every mouthful count in nutritional value. In spite of this, however, it is common especially in retirement homes, for elderly people to be fed on cream and rich puddings, which ruin their chances of health and vitality.

Of course, as with any diet, if you've had health problems in the past you must talk to your doctor before you start on the Moerman diet.

Since the eight substances that form the foundation of the Moerman diet are all easily available from the chemist as tablets, you might wonder whether you could just take the tablets, instead of following the diet. The answer is that vitamin and mineral pills can never replace natural foods.

This is because fruit, cereals and vegetables always contain a combination of vitamins, minerals, acids and fruit sugars which help the body break down and digest the food, and absorb the valuable ingredients. Cereals and rice, or potatoes, for example, naturally contain special enzymes. These are chemicals which work to break down food. There are many different enzymes, and each works on a different kind of food. Natural, wholegrain foods contain all the enzymes you need to digest them.

Modern refining methods, however, remove some of the vitamins and enzymes, so the food becomes harder for the body to digest and use. For this reason you should always eat brown rice, and use grains and cereals that have been processed as little as possible.

9

The Moerman Diet

The Moerman diet is designed to strengthen the immune system, so the body can fight disease naturally. It allows you to choose each day between the permitted foods, and some menus and recipe suggestions are given later in the book. But you must *not eat anything* that isn't included, as the diet is carefully worked out to include all the eight vital substances, and other foods can strip them from the body.

YOU MAY EAT AND DRINK

- Buttermilk – at least a pint a day, or alternate with Quark (thickened sour milk, available from supermarkets)
- Wholemeal bread – see page 51 for recipe. Eat it with butter, or cottage cheese.
- Egg yolks – two a day for adults, one for children, but not egg whites. Patients suffering from liver or gall diseases should not eat egg yolk at first.
- Vegetable juice, especially beetroot juice, which removes toxins, and carrot juice.
- Fruit juice – three lemons a day, diluted with orange juice if you like, or try apple or pear juice. All fruit juice should be freshly made, and must *never* be sweetened with sugar.
- Brown rice, either boiled in water as it is or ground and cooked in milk.

- Vegetables, especially raw ones. Lettuce, cucumber, tomatoes, radishes, paprika, carrots, chicory and beetroot are all excellent. Cooked vegetables such as carrots, green beans, spinach, beetroot and asparagus are also good, although some vitamins and minerals are always lost in cooking. Occasionally, cauliflower, parsley, brussels sprouts and green cabbage can be eaten.
- Fruit is excellent, and you should eat as much as you can. The only prohibited fruits are rhubarb, dates, figs and sweet grapes. Oranges, apples, pears, plums, apricots and peaches are all good, and so are dried fruits, such as plums, apricots and raisins, although these should first be soaked in water for 24 hours.
- Fruit and vegetables should be prepared and cooked as little as possible, using no sugar and very little salt. Organic vegetables, which have been grown without artificial fertilizer and haven't been sprayed with chemicals, are definitely the best.
- You may eat some black pepper, a little nutmeg, pure honey (1 teaspoon a day), cold pressed olive or sunflower oil (do not heat), cream every now and then, and homemade porridge, made with wheat flakes, barley, oatflakes etc, and eaten with milk, is very nutritious.

YOU MAY *NOT* EAT OR DRINK

- Meat, fish or poultry, including stocks and broths, and all shellfish.
- Coffee, tea or cocoa.

- Sugar of any kind, or any food containing sugar – sweets, cakes, chocolate etc.
- White flour, or anything made with it – white bread, cakes, biscuits, pasta or puddings.
- Any animal fat – lard, bacon fat etc., except butter.
- All margarines and heat-pressed vegetable oils.
- Anything fried or baked.
- Yoghurt
- Fizzy drinks or squashes
- Alcohol
- White cabbage
- Celery
- Rhubarb
- Pulses – lentils, kidney beans, split peas, haricot beans, soya beans, etc.
- Potatoes, because they contain carbohydrates which are difficult to digest.
- Mushrooms
- All artificial colourings and preservatives
- Smoking is absolutely forbidden. It is the most important known cause of lung cancer, and it also causes several other kinds of cancer, and other serious diseases such as heart attacks. There is no point in following the Moerman diet if you smoke at the same time.

By following these guidelines you can try the Moerman diet for yourself. The three golden rules are:

- Chew your food well
- Never eat more than you want
- Prepare everything carefully, so the food doesn't lose vitamins and minerals

Vitamin supplements

Vitamin supplements are a valuable addition to the diet. Everyone can take vitamin C tablets, although if you suffer from stomach or liver complaints, or high blood pressure, you should take your doctor's advice first. The tablets can be bought at any chemist, but you should avoid the effervescent sort, which fizz when you dissolve them in water, or lemon-flavoured ones, as both may contain harmful chemicals. If you haven't taken vitamin C before, start with a low dose and build up gradually.

Daily doses of vitamin C

Adults	Up to 1250 mg each day	
Children	Depending on age:	
	up to 4 years	250 mg per day
	up to 8 years	500 mg per day
	up to 12 years	750 mg per day
	up to 16 years	1000 mg per day

Never take the tablets on an empty stomach, and always dissolve them in buttermilk, vegetable or fruit juices.

You should talk to your doctor about taking supplements of vitamins A, B complex, E, and iron. You may need to take a multi-vitamin every day, but if you take supplements of only one vitamin you may be upsetting your body's natural balance. If you take just B6, for example, you will reduce your store of the other B vitamins.

How To Use The Diet

A typical day's menu on the Moerman diet could be something like this:

Breakfast	The juice of 2 oranges and a lemon Wholemeal bread with butter and cheese Buttermilk
Mid-morning	Beetroot juice with lemon, fruit
Lunch	Rice cooked with vegetables Mixed salad Quark Fruit
Mid-afternoon	Buttermilk with grape juice Fruit
Supper	Pea soup Wholemeal bread Buttermilk
Late evening	Buttermilk with orange and lemon juice Warm milk before you go to bed

You can vary the menu as much as you like, within the rules of the Moerman diet. For example, you might have muesli with milk instead of bread and cheese for breakfast.

Variety

To put a bit of variety into the diet, why not try some of these ideas?

Drinks

- Mix buttermilk with oranges or lemon juice, or try adding strawberrries, grated apple or egg yolk
- Beetroot juice mixes nicely with equal quantities of lemon juice and buttermilk
- Try carrot juice with diced pineapple
- Put some diced pineapple (fresh, not tinned) into the liquidizer with apple or lemon juice and buttermilk. Whizz it all up for a pineapple milk-shake.
- Make a nourishing grapefruit drink with the juice of one grapefruit and one orange, and two egg yolks.
- Try adding some grape juice to this recipe, with honey to sweeten it if you like.
- Mix some ripe tomatoes, some celeriac, an onion and some carrots in the blender, and drink as fresh as possible!

Good healthy bread is essential for the Moerman diet. You can buy good wholewheat bread from health food shops and some supermarkets, or why not make your own, so you know exactly what's in it?

Wholemeal bread

1½ lb/750 g wholemeal flour
3 teaspoons dried yeast, or 6 tsp fresh
1 teaspoon sea salt
¾ pint/450 ml lukewarm milk
honey

Mix the flour and the salt. Dissolve the yeast in half the milk, mixed with some honey, and wait until it has a good frothy head on it. Then add to the flour, with the remaining milk. Mix thoroughly, and then knead well for a good five minutes. Put the dough in a warm place, and leave it until it has doubled in size (about 1–2 hours). Then knead again, and put it into a buttered bread tin. Leave to rise in the tin for about half an hour.

Bake at 200 C/400 F/Gas mark 6 for 40 minutes, until the loaf sounds hollow when you knock on the bottom. Be careful not to let it bake too brown, though.

You can vary the recipe by adding extra ingredients to the dough. For example:

- 8 oz/200 g raisins
- 2 chopped apples and 4 oz/100 g raisins
- 4 chopped apples and a little cinnamon
- 8 oz/200 g shredded apricots

Spreads and toppings for bread

Cream cheese and hard cheese can be eaten in moderate amounts. There are lots of different kinds of cheese without salt and with a low fat content available in supermarkets, so it shouldn't be difficult to find one you like. Mild cheeses are better than matured kinds.

For a basic spread, mix 1 oz/25 g butter with 4 oz/100 g grated cheese. Add an egg yolk and 2 tablespoons milk or cream, and blend it all together.

You could try adding:

- Coarsely ground hazelnuts
- A chopped tomato
- Some pieces of pineapple
- 3 tablespoons chutney
- Chopped leeks, or celeriac, or parsley, or onions. . . .

Or you could try one of these toppings:

- 4 oz/100 g quark, mixed with the juice of half a lemon, some grated radishes and some chopped celeriac
- 4 oz/100 g sour cream, spring onions and herbs
- Cress, sprinkled with lemon juice and topped with thin slices of tomato

SOUPS

Vegetable soups are easy to prepare, and make a tasty, nourishing meal.

Pea soup

½ lb/250 g green peas with pods
1 stick celery
2 onions
2 pints/1 litre vegetable broth (see page 55)

Bring the vegetables to the boil in the broth, and simmer for 15 minutes.

For variety you could add

- Celeriac
- Carrots
- Leeks
- Basil or thyme for flavour

Tomato soup

6 tomatoes
1½ pints/¾ litre water
1 vegetable stock cube
1 tablespoon wheat flakes
Chopped celeriac, parsley and onion

Peel and chop the tomatoes. Bring the water to the boil and add the stock cube and the wheat flakes. Then add the tomatoes and the other vegetables, and bring to the boil briefly.

Leek soup

1 onion, chopped
White parts of 2 leeks, sliced finely
1 oz/50 g buckwheat
Bayleaf
1 egg yolk

Heat the onion, leeks, buckwheat and bayleaf gently in
1¼ pints/¾ litre water, and allow to simmer for 20
minutes. Remove from the heat and take out the
bayleaf. Beat the egg yolk and add it to the soup,
swirling the liquid as the egg cooks.

Cauliflower soup

½ cauliflower
1 pint/½ litre milk
4 oz/100 g wholemeal flour
1 vegetable stock cube
2 egg yolks

Boil the cauliflower in water for 15 minutes. Then
remove from the pan, and break into chunks. Add the
milk, stock cube and flour, mixed to a paste with a little
water, to the water in the pan. Bring to the boil, and then
return the cauliflower to the pan. Remove from the heat,
and add the egg yolks. Serve with grated cheese and a
pinch of nutmeg.

THE MOERMAN DIET

Cucumber soup

1 cucumber, diced
5 tomatoes, peeled and chopped
1 onion, chopped

Boil the vegetables in vegetable stock, or water with a
vegetable stock cube, for about 15 minutes. Allow to
cool a little, then add a handful of grated cheese and let it
melt through.

Vegetable broth

1 onion
2 carrots
White part of 1 leek
Celeriac
1 tomato
1 pepper, red or green
parsley
Bay leaf

Chop the vegetables roughly, and bring to the boil in 2
pints/1 litre water. Allow to simmer for an hour, then
strain.

Vegetables

Fresh vegetables lie at the heart of the Moerman diet. They are a valuable source of vitamins and minerals, and contain the enzymes which are so central to the healing process.

Not all vegetables are permitted under the Moerman diet. You should avoid red and white cabbage, and sauerkraut in particular, and rhubarb can also be harmful. But you can make the most of the others. They're full of fibre, and so they'll give you energy without making you fat. Organic vegetables are best, of course, because they've been grown without harmful fertilisers and chemicals. You might even try growing your own!

Try and eat vegetables in season, so you know they haven't been 'forced' in greenhouses, as this can strip them of vital nutrients. Here are some suggestions for seasonal vegetables.

Spring
Chicory, asparagus, cauliflower, broccoli, peas, cucumber, lettuce, turnips, leeks, radishes, spinach, green beans, cress.

Summer
Aubergines, beetroot, celeriac, peppers, tomatoes, onions, turnips, and many of the spring and salad vegetables.

Autumn
Brussel sprouts, green cabbage, carrots, chicory.

Winter
Chicory, endives, beetroots, turnips and parsnips.

Cooking and preparation of vegetables

You should always boil vegetables in as little water as you can, while preventing them from sticking or burning, and with little or no salt. Boil them for just as long as they need, to avoid destroying vitamins. When you get used to it you'll agree that most vegetables taste better if they've still got a bit of 'bite' in them.

Salads

Salads made from raw vegetables have a vital role to play in the Moerman diet. You can use your imagination to give variety, and serve the salad as a starter, to eat with your meal, or afterwards with cheese instead of a dessert.

Green salad

Wash the lettuce leaves as usual, and make a dressing from the juice of two lemons, instead of vinegar, and sunflower oil.

To liven up a green salad you could add:

- grated beetroot and apple
- grated carrot and paprika
- some finely chopped chicory
- cucumber and tomato
- carrots and radishes
- diced apple, parsley and horse-radish
- endive or spinach

Summer salad

Cold rice
1 large cucumber
tomatoes
1 shredded onion
garden herbs
celeriac
chopped peppers

Chop all the ingredients roughly and mix with the juice of two lemons and 4 tablespoons of sunflower oil. Let it settle for a while, so all the flavours can blend together, and serve chilled.

Salad dressings

All salads cry out for dressing. Home-made mayonnaise, made with egg yolks, is a good basis, and you could add any of the following for variety:

- parsley
- a finely chopped onion
- chopped celeriac
- chopped pepper, green or red
- 1 tablespoon lemon juice
- 2 tablespoons orange juice

Rice

As potatoes and pasta aren't permitted on the Moerman diet rice will become a very important ingredient in your meals. You should never eat white rice, as the process of cleaning and refining it strips out all the goodness. Instead buy natural brown rice, which you can find in most supermarkets, or in health food stores.

Rice is very rich in nutrients. In fact, it's about as close to 'the perfect food' as you could hope to find for providing all the elements you need in your diet. A helping of rice contains protein, fats (especially the valuable unsaturated fats), carbohydrates, sodium, potassium, calcium, phosphorous, magnesium, iron, fluoride, vitamins E, B1 and B2.

In general you only need one cup of rice per person. Each cupful needs to cook in two cups of water, and you should always add the rice to the water when it is boiling. It takes about 45 minutes to cook, but there are now 'quick-cook' varieties available, which take about 20 minutes. As a final touch you can add chopped celeriac, leek or onions.

Rice and peas

Cook equal quantities of rice and peas (or you can use yesterday's leftovers). Mix them together, and add a little butter.

You could add:

- a little vegetable broth, for seasoning
- a few fresh herbs
- spinach
- tomatoes
- some grated cheese

Rice also makes an ideal accompaniment to all other main meals.

MAIN MEALS

Pizza

Make a pizza base with wholewheat flour, and top it with tomatoes, cheese, chopped celeriac, parsley, or anything else you fancy!

Vegetable stew

Beans, chicory, cauliflower, peas, turnips and other vegetables make a very good stew. Cook in the oven with a little water or broth and some herbs, and serve with grated cheese.

SAUCES

Onion Sauce

Bring to the boil 1 litre/2 pints water containing vegetable broth. Add 1 or 2 chopped onions, and let it boil for 5 minutes.

Mix 2 tablespoons of cornflour with a little water, and add it to the sauce to thicken it. Then let the sauce cool a little, and add 2 tablespoons sunflower oil.

You can vary this sauce by adding grated cheese, a handful of parsley, some chopped celeriac, or finely shredded pepper, with the oil.

Tomato Sauce

Peel and chop 4 tomatoes, and boil them for 5 minutes in ½ litre/1 pint water, with a chopped onion and some vegetable broth. Thicken with rice or wholemeal flour, and add some sunflower oil as the sauce cools. You could also add some cheese or two egg yolks.

DESSERTS

Having read (and cooked) your way through the diet so far you'll see that, with a little imagination, your meals needn't be restricted by the limitations of the diet. You'll probably find you're even enjoying it, and in the end that's what matters most – your health and the enjoyment you get from life. And desserts in particular should be fun to prepare and to eat, so here are some suggestions.

Strawberry cocktail

Mix some strawberries with diced apples, pears, cherries and any other fruit in season, and drench with unsweetened apple juice.

Melon bowl

Mix finely diced melon, apples and pears, with unsweetened grape juice. Serve chilled.

Fruit bread

Bake your wholewheat bread in the usual way, but try adding apples or raisins to the mixture.

Cooked pears

Peel and halve the pears, and remove the cores. Bake them in the oven with a little water and a pinch of cinnamon.

10

New Support for
Dr Moerman

In Copenhagen in 1906 three rats were caught in a sugar refinery, and were found to be suffering from stomach disease. They were brought to the laboratory of the noted Danish pathologist Dr Fibiger, who examined them, and found that a parasitic worm had burrowed through the stomach of each of the rats, and the stomach cells around the worm in each case showed signs of being abnormal. He had them examined by several independent pathologists, who all came to the same conclusion – the rats had cancer of the stomach, and this was in some way caused by the worm. The worm itself is quite a common parasite in rats, as it spends part of its life as a grub inside the bodies of cockroaches. When rats eat the cockroaches they absorb the grubs as well, and they grow to be adult worms inside the rats.

In scientific circles Dr Fibiger's discovery was welcomed with great enthusiasm, as it seemed to serve as evidence to back up the theories about cancer that were fashionable at the time, that all cancers are caused by some kind of long-term irritation in the body.

In 1926 Dr Fibiger received a Nobel prize for his work. Unfortunately, a few years later the cause of the cancer in these rats was shown to be not the parasitic worm, but a lack of vitamin A in the rats' diet. In 1951 the Dutch Cancer Institute carried out his experiments again, but this time the rats didn't get cancer.

At a conference in the same year the director of the Dutch Cancer Institute asked Dr Moerman why this should be. Dr Moerman's reply was that in the Dutch experiment the rats must have been fed a balanced diet, so they were able to withstand the invasion of a cancer. He explained the importance of the balanced diet by suggesting that certain substances had the capacity to 'melt away' cancer cells and tumours, and although modern science had not yet been able to identify exactly what they were he predicted that they would be found to be one of his vital eight substances.

He was proved right in both these predictions. When Dr Fibiger's experiments were compared in detail with those done in Holland, where the rats *didn't* get cancer, it was seen that the rats in Copenhagen were fed bread mixed with water, but the Dutch rats had their food mixed with milk. Milk contains vitamin A, and it was the shortage of this vitamin, not the parasitic worm, which caused Dr Fibiger's results.

Of course, Dr Moerman didn't dismiss the idea that the parasitic worm had played a role in causing cancer in the rats that were found to have it. His point was that the emphasis he placed on it was very different. Dr Fibiger and his associates thought that they had somehow proved that Dr Moerman and those who were working along the same lines were wrong, because the worm was what caused the cancer, but Dr Moerman demonstrated that the really crucial difference between the rats that got cancer and those that didn't lay in their capacity to *resist* infection, which depended on their diet.

To this day doctors and scientists are interested in researching which irritant factors trigger off cancers, although nowadays they concentrate on factors such as viruses. But what interested Dr Moerman more, and what continues to be researched and investigated in the search for a cure, was the idea that the body can be reinforced so that there are no weakened potential cancer cells for the trigger factors to work on.

In 1983, 77 years after the Copenhagen experiments, Dr Moerman's other prediction was backed up by another series of experiments, this time carried out by another doctor at the Dutch Cancer Institute. He demonstrated that there are certain substances which help the body fight off cancers, and he gave them the name 'anti-carcinogens'. When Dr Moerman produced his explanations this word didn't exist, but when he talked about substances which could 'melt away' tumours he was describing the same process.

The anti-carcinogens work on the DNA of the cancer cells and alter their genetic structure, which is the root of what makes them so dangerous to the body. But they work in an indirect way, by stopping the build-up of harmful enzymes in the cancerous cells.

This evidence provided valuable scientific support for Dr Moerman's work, because the research identified vitamin A and its derivatives, particularly retinol, as important anti-carcinogens. Under a microscope the Dutch researchers saw that vitamin A could not only slow the growth of a cancer tumour, but in some cases it could turn a malignant tumour into a benign (harmless) one.

The biotechnology industry, especially the American companies which are in the forefront of this research, are very interested in investigating the possibilities for using anti-carcinogens and restricting enzymes to find a cure for cancer. At Johns Hopkins University, which makes a speciality of this kind of research, young biotechnologists are brought on fast to meet the ever-increasing demand for their skills. The industry is growing at 25 per cent every year, and 5000 jobs are already waiting.

In the parallel research into the trigger factors, which cause cancer in people whose immune systems are below par, researchers in the US have recently become interested in the role of nutrition. A recent study has shown that 35 per cent of cases of cancer in the US can be traced to diet, especially a diet high in fat (there is a high risk of breast cancer, for example, with a very fatty diet), 30 per cent can be attributed to smoking (lung cancer), 3 per cent to alcohol and heavy drinking, 3 per cent to natural radioactivity in the environment, 2 per cent to pollution and 1 per cent to taking certain medicines. In addition 4 per cent could be linked to what are known as 'occupational risks', such as contact with asbestos and vinyl chloride, which can cause testicular cancer. This can be greatly helped nowadays using hormone preparation, and the results are encouraging, although these drugs do have side-effects such as vomiting, and they need constant kidney dilation to prevent serious damage to the kidneys.

More research has been carried out recently, especially at the Vitamin Research Institute in Bad Soden, in Germany, about the effects of pollution of the ozone layer, which is constantly in the news. The ozone layer in the earth's atmosphere protects the earth from harmful rays of the sun. This precious layer is destroyed by chemicals known as CFCs, which are found in everyday aerosol sprays and polystyrene packaging, like the packets used by hamburger chains. Without its protection dangerous radioactive rays can reach our skin. They build up in our bodies, and damage cell walls and prevent natural enzymes from working properly.

This new research shows that vitamins A, C and E can neutralize the effects of these rays, and help protect our bodies against them. The doses the researchers recommend are, like Dr Moerman's, quite high – they suggest doses of vitamin A two or three times the normal requirement, and up to 10 times the doses for vitamins C and E. These high doses have been shown to protect the body against lung, stomach and intestinal cancers. In patients suffering from these cancers the levels of these vitamins in the blood are always low, so large quantities are necessary.

So whether you take the opinion of the National Cancer Research Council of the USA, the Institute for Vitamin Research or the Dutch Cancer Institute again and again, however indirectly, the ideas of Dr Moerman are backed up: where cancer is the result of a bad diet it can be healed. And whatever the scepticism of some doctors, the message is getting through to ordinary people. In surveys of popular opinion more and more people are saying again and again that what they want is healing, not more remedies and drug treatments. So Dr Moerman really was fifty years ahead of his time!

Different sorts of cancer

There are over a hundred different cancers. They can be

caused by a disease, such as a virus, by CFCs and their effect on the environment, by other dangerous chemicals or by contact with radioactive substances in the environment. The one thing they all have in common is that when someone gets cancer it's always because their immune system is weakened, and can't withstand the invasion.

Apart from tumours there are also cancers known as 'malignant system diseases'. These have their source not in the tissue of the body but in the bone marrow, and they include diseases such as leukaemia. They show up in a huge increase in the number of underdeveloped white blood cells, which indicate that the white blood cells aren't able to mature properly and work as part of the immune system. What they have in common with tumours is the characteristic way the cells grow and multiply.

New developments to treat these cancers are concentrating on substances called zytostatics. These are chemicals which control the growth of cells in the body, and so help stop the spread of diseases such as leukaemia and Hodgkinson's disease in the body. Some of these substances are found in nature – they are produced by mustard plants and meadow saffron – and others have been produced in the laboratory. They have been shown to be quite effective in controlling tumours, and don't have such serious side-effects as the drugs traditionally used in chemotherapy, but they can't help strengthen the immune system or help the body fight back on its own. So they can be useful as a short-term measure against a tumour, but in the long term only a cure which restores the whole body can help it heal itself the natural way.

11

Conclusion

Mrs Maat had a tumour in her intestines. She had an operation but the tumour soon returned, and the secondary tumours spread so fast that her doctor advised her that a second operation was useless. He referred her to Dr Moerman, though, as a last hope. Two years later he could note on her medical records that she was perfectly well.

Mrs van Oeveren had cancer of the stomach. When she first came for an appointment with Dr Moerman she'd lost so much weight that she was dangerously thin. Her doctor said he could operate to remove the tumour, but not the many secondary tumours which had spread all round her body. She began to follow the Moerman diet and take the vitamin supplements, and immediately she began to put on weight. She recovered, and went on to live a full and healthy life.

The world of orthodox medicine couldn't ignore success stories like these for ever. The proof was there for all to see, in the patients he cured. It took a long time, but the doctors had to admit in the end that it's the cure that counts.

Dr Moerman's years of devoted and painstaking research hold out new hope of a cure for people everywhere. People who had been resigned to despair now have confident hope for the future. His methods have cured many hundreds, and the number of 'Moerman doctors' is growing every day. These men and women don't just pay lip service to the theory, they put it into practice every day, and the positive vitality on the face of each patient they discharge tells them their faith is justified.

The combination of diet, supplement therapy and the patients' own determination gives us a whole new approach to the problem of cancer. It is no longer the remorseless invading force, everyone's darkest fear. Now it can be beaten, and you can win.

Useful Addresses

If you'd like to know more about using the Dr Moerman cancer diet, or you'd like to contact one of the Moerman doctors, there is an organization in Holland run specially for Moerman doctors and their patients. It was set up in 1974 by a Dutch woman after Dr Moerman cured her 11-year-old son, who was suffering from a brain tumour. Amnestie gives advice about doctors and new treatments and diets, and can put patients in touch with one another to give each other help and support. They produce a bulletin six times a year, giving the latest news about cancer treatment. You can contact them at:

Amnestie
PO Box 14
NL–6673 ZG Andelst
Netherlands

Amnestie has over ten thousand members. It will be able to put you in touch with one of the Moerman doctors, who all speak English.

The Bristol Cancer Help Centre has used elements of Dr Moerman's diet. You can contact them at:

Cancer Help Centre
Grove House
Cornwallis Grove
Clifton
Bristol BS8 4PG
0272 743216

Another body concerned with alternative therapies for cancer is:

New Approaches to Cancer
Addington Park
Maidstone
Kent ME19 5BL
0732 848336

Index